Dr. Mao's
Harmony

Tai Chi

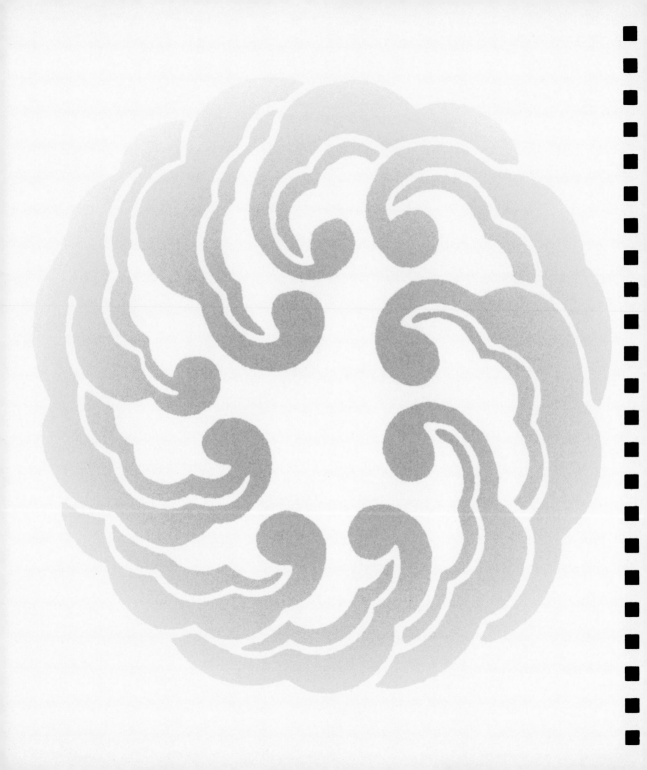

Dr. Mao's
Harmony

Tai Chi

Simple Practice for Health and Well-Being

by Dr. Maoshing Ni

illustrations by Nicole Kaufman

CHRONICLE BOOKS

SAN FRANCISCO

Library of Congress Cataloging-in-Publication Data:

Ni, Maoshing.
    Dr. Mao's Harmony Tai chi : simple practice for health and well-being /
    by Maoshing Ni.
    p. cm.
    ISBN-13: 978-0-8118-4950-0
    ISBN-10: 0-8118-4950-3
1. Tai chi   I. Title.
    GV504.N55 2006
    613.7'148—dc22   2005030703

Manufactured in China

Designed by Laurie Dolphin Design
Design Implementation by folio2

Distributed in Canada by Raincoast Books
9050 Shaughnessy Street
Vancouver, British Columbia V6P 6E5

10 9 8 7 6 5 4 3 2 1

Chronicle Books LLC
85 Second Street
San Francisco, California 94105

www.chroniclebooks.com

*acknowledg*ments

The genesis of this book actually began with my collaboration with Dr. Joseph Miller, whose efforts in compiling my father's and my previous works on tai chi form the foundation of this book. As director of the Chi Health Institute and a professor at UCLA Medical School, his dedication to transmitting the art and benefits of my family's harmony tai chi tradition is highly commendable and much valued.

Without my father's disciplined instructions while growing up in Asia, I would not have become proficient in tai chi, nor would I have developed an appreciation for movement arts as a tool for health, happiness, and spiritual development. I am forever indebted to him, for he is the source of both my knowledge and inspiration.

I am deeply appreciative to Laurie Dolphin, my collaborator, whose design talents are abundantly and pleasingly displayed throughout the book. Many thanks to Laurie's assistant, Allison Meierding, whose tireless assistance in the descriptive wordings of the movements helped to make them easier to follow.

I am grateful to Jodi Davis, our editor at Chronicle Books, who believed in us and supported our vision for an essential and easy-to-learn book on tai chi. I am thankful for her patience and assistance in making this book a reality. Also thanks go to her assistant, Kate Prouty, for keeping everything in order and on track.

Special thanks go to Mark Johnson, whose years of experience in teaching tai chi to Westerners made him well suited to polish the original text into its present form.

I am so happy and thankful to Nicole Kaufman for illustrating the movements within this book. It is truly an art form to be able to render the drawings accurately for ease of learning.

I appreciate my wife, Emm, and our children, Yu-Shien Michelle, Yu-Shing Natasha, and Yu-Kai Nicholas, for their support and understanding. They are part of the purpose for this book. I thank my brother and longtime partner, Dr. Daoshing Ni, and his wife, Tracy, for their unwavering commitment and support of our family tradition.

Finally, I am beholden to all of my tai chi students, associates, researchers, and practitioners, and to teachers of tai chi everywhere, for their dedication in spreading the art and benefits of tai chi so that even more people can enjoy health, wellness, and peace throughout the world.

Contents

*intro*duction

Tai chi is a sequence of slow, meditative movements, a hybrid of yoga and martial arts based on the cyclical movements of the natural world. Unlike spiritual traditions that ask us to renounce our daily lives, tai chi promises us a more harmonious connection to our familiar routines. Its goal is simple: to reconnect us to the flow of energy that permeates the entire universe. When that energy becomes truly available to us, our vitality is boundless.

In Chinese, *tai chi* literally means "infinity." It is part of the family of *qi* arts, each one designed to help us unblock and strengthen our internal energy. Qi (pronounced chē), "energy" or "vital force," is the principle that animates the entire universe, from the microscopic to the galactic level. When our qi flows without blockage or interruption, we enjoy boundless health and vitality. Tai chi is a gentle yet effective path to allowing that healing energy to flow freely.

Practicing tai chi is exceedingly easy. Its ancient wisdom is not revealed by studying complicated concepts or practicing joyless physical discipline. It is less an exercise than a gentle celebration of life itself. Each movement of tai chi reflects and expresses cosmic balance.

Various traditions and styles of tai chi have been developed and handed down through many generations. Today, the Yang, Chen, Wu, Hao, and Sun styles are the most common, and numerous books, magazine articles, and Web sites are devoted to them.

This book explores a style of tai chi called Harmony Tai Chi, which distills the essence of the Chen, Yang, and Wu styles. The Chen style, one of China's oldest, originated as a martial art and is quite dynamic. The Yang style emphasizes slow, expansive movements. The Wu style moves from a smaller stance than the other styles. Thus, the study of Harmony Tai Chi allows the student to combine the grace and tranquility of one school with the dynamism and agility of the others. It allows the student to experience the interplay of yin and yang energies and become attuned to the harmonious rhythms that animate the natural world.

In addition to six basic stances, this book delineates eighteen foundation exercises that can be completed in fifteen to twenty minutes and will provide an unparalleled experience for both the body and the spirit.

How Does **Harmony Tai Chi** Differ from Other Forms?

Harmony Tai Chi differs from ordinary Tai Chi Chuan in that it more fully implements and emphasizes the principles contained in Lao Tzu's *Tao Te Ching* (or, the *Way of Life*) and the *I Ching* (or, the *Book of Changes and Unchanging Truth*). Harmony Tai Chi originated from the Integral Way spiritual tradition of ancient China, which is known for preserving and distilling the essence of wisdom through the ages. This tradition and its teaching are being carried on by the Ni family in the West. Since Harmony Tai Chi has a balanced focus on integrating the body, mind, and spirit, it is the style most accessible to men and women of any age.

The purpose of the Eighteen-Step Harmony Tai Chi Form is to provide an opportunity for students new to Harmony Tai Chi or tai chi in general to experience the joy and spiritual uplift offered by this unique style. It introduces some of the basic movements of the full 108-Posture Harmony Tai Chi Long Form, and it is a style easily learned by anyone interested in improving his or her health and well-being. It also can be used profitably as a daily practice. With movements such as "Empty, Yet Productive," "Move without Exhaustion," "Within There Is Essence," and "Exposition of the Heavenly Mystery," Harmony Tai Chi embodies the same principles taught in the various chapters of the *Tao Te Ching*. Harmony Tai Chi is like the rhythmic dance of the four seasons—sprouting, expanding, harvesting, and returning to the root—a dance that endlessly renews itself.

The Origins of Tai Chi

The principle or philosophy of tai chi started simply. Approximately ten thousand years ago, people in China began to closely observe the cycles of nature, eventually developing a series of movements based on the dynamic patterns of the natural world. Tai chi is one of the most popular of these systems of self-awareness and physical development. Based on the recognition that our bodies are like miniature universes, the gentle movements of tai chi attune our inner energy flow to the flow of nature itself. As nature so dramatically demonstrates, we've got to keep moving!

But tai chi is far more than a sport or a dance. By practicing tai chi, we transform ideas into actual physical experience. Feeling how energy circulates through our bodies as we practice the movements of tai chi, we become intimate with the laws of the universe. Doing tai chi means balancing ourselves physically, emotionally, and spiritually. In tai chi we move, but gently enough to preserve our inner calm and composure. The subtle energy of our mind and spirit merges with the coarser energy of our body.

Tai Chi Is Everything

The integration of yin and yang is called tai chi. Passive and active, day and night, hot and cold: when opposites are harmonized, we achieve balance.

Everything that exists is an expression of tai chi. Every small particle is a tai chi. The vast universe is a tai chi. The gathering of small events or units is a tai chi. The dispersion of the vast universe is a tai chi. There is nothing beyond tai chi or excluded from it. Thus, the individual body is a tai chi. The cosmic body is also a tai chi. Tai Chi is the integral truth of the Universe.

From the *Hua Hu Ching*

In tai chi we are not merely striving to achieve precise physical movements. We are learning the secrets of physical health and longevity by participating in the cycles of energy that flow through the universe. All life consists of cycles; even the energies of the human organism circulate through the body. Our practice of tai chi reminds us that linear movement always comes to an end. Tai chi teaches us to transform a straight line of energy into a circle, putting us in touch with never-ending energy. Everything in the universe tends to follow a circular pattern. The earth spins on its axis as it orbits the sun. The sun, in turn, orbits the galactic center of the Milky Way. The galaxy itself forms a circular pattern as it courses through the universe. All of the movements of tai chi are a series of circles, which reflect this eternal cosmic law.

The Fundamental **Principles** of Tai Chi

Undivided oneness, or *wu chi*, is the origin of every manifestation in the universe. It is the unshakable stillness at the core of tai chi, the background and foundation for the dynamic play of energy, or *qi*. As this primal qi energy moves, it has a polarizing effect, creating yin and yang, light and dark, feminine and masculine, left and right, and so on. The dynamic interactions of these polarities account for the endless variety of the physical world—which, for all its diversity, is still fundamentally one. Through our practice of tai chi, we gain a visceral knowledge of this unity amid diversity.

The practice of tai chi trains the mind to observe the body in every detail. In this way, rather than scattering energy through mindless physical activity, we gather and retain it. The peaceful mental atmosphere created by tai chi movement helps negative thought patterns to dissolve and be replaced by positive, life-enhancing attitudes.

By learning tai chi movement, we can remedy our incompleteness and energy imbalance. Tai chi accomplishes this without dogma or a rigid belief system. It improves our personalities by refining and harmonizing our yin and yang energies, resulting in an even temperament and calm disposition. These qualities enable us to remain poised even in the most difficult situations. After all, to be excessively positive or negative is ultimately madness. Only by harmonizing the dualities in our mind can we achieve the balance that brings peace.

What Is **Qi**?

Qi energy circulates continuously through the channels of our bodies, not unlike the way water flows in a riverbed. But most people's qi is weak, pooled and stagnating in cavities instead of powerfully flowing. Our minds can influence the circulation of qi. The more we train our minds and our qi, the more responsive and powerful they become. Ultimately, when the mind and qi are in concert, we enjoy harmony and health. When the mind and qi are at cross-purposes, there is chaos and disease.

In tai chi, we learn movements that both contract and expand qi energy. We simultaneously send it out and reel it in. This flow of opposites is the dance of yin and yang.

The Principles of **Yin and Yang**

Yin and yang are the opposing poles of all things. In nature, these opposite aspects complement one another. Summer's heat and light are counterbalanced by winter's cold and dark. Vigorous activity is followed by rest. What goes up must come down. Even our bodies have a top (yang) and a bottom (yin). We have a left side that is yang and a right side that is yin.

In tai chi there is a continual sequence of yin and yang movements. An upward movement will be balanced by a downward movement. A gesture with the left side will be complemented by a gesture with the right side. The inhalation and exhalation of our breath also reflects the symmetry of yin and yang.

The Principle of **Integration**

Some forms of exercise engage only a limited number of muscles. In tai chi, every aspect of our bodies is involved—not just the muscles, but also the nervous, digestive, respiratory, and endocrine systems. Sports and many common exercise routines often cause rapid, shallow breathing, which strains the heart and lungs. Tai chi's deep, slow breathing coaxes more oxygen into the bloodstream, warming and strengthening the internal organs. As we practice tai chi, every aspect of our bodies is gradually strengthened, developed, and refined.

Tai chi is a moving meditation. It cultivates stillness in the midst of movement and dynamic energy in the midst of stillness. It helps us integrate and unify what seem to be opposites. Chinese ancestors observed how stillness and movement continually follow each other. Movement is yang, stillness is yin. If we merely sit and meditate, we risk letting our vital energy stagnate. To benefit from quiet meditation, we must balance it with smooth, flowing activity. Abrupt movement, however, also causes energy to stagnate, because it exhausts us. It's as if we tried to sprint full speed to a distant place: we would soon get tired and collapse. Walking at a relaxed pace, we would arrive at our destination still raring to go. Smooth, rhythmic, flowing movements help energy flow and can be sustained indefinitely.

The Principle of **Regeneration**

Another essential principle of tai chi movement is that we never extend our bodies completely. We always keep some energy in reserve. We go as far as a certain point and then return to the center to regroup our forces. By practicing this principle, the student of tai chi enjoys the possibility of continual self-regeneration. Everything in nature follows a cyclical process of growth and evolution. All things grow and develop, and after their peak has been reached, they revert back to their source to regenerate again. We might say that nature's energy is constantly recycled.

Tai Chi as **Martial Art**

Tai chi trains the body and mind to function as one. It fosters calmness and self-control, even during times of extreme duress. Those who pursue tai chi as a martial art find that it helps them to defend themselves in a controlled and balanced manner, without fear or anger. Even those who practice tai chi simply for health find it useful when they are called upon to defend themselves.

We are all affected by our surroundings. We become disappointed or upset when our plans fail. We are annoyed by the carelessness or ill will of others. Sometimes we respond impatiently, without thought or consideration. In practicing tai chi we learn not to fight, but to yield. Even when attacked, we can use calm movement to transform the situation. If we allow ourselves to move gracefully, we can keep a challenging situation from escalating.

Harmony Tai Chi approaches tai chi not as a martial art, but as an ancient spiritual tradition. However, sometimes this book will refer to martial-arts principles to help students better understand a movement. Tai chi is an effective method of self-defense, but its essential value is as a philosophical and spiritual practice.

The Healing **Benefits** of Tai Chi

Ideally, our energy regenerates as it circulates through our body. But in ordinary exercise, a lot of energy is squandered through overheating and perspiration. In tai chi we avoid overexertion. Tai chi is a self-healing practice that can be enjoyed by anyone regardless of age, fitness, or state of health. The therapeutic aspects of tai chi, long recognized in China, have only recently been acknowledged in the West. Consistent practice of tai chi balances our internal energies so effectively that it has been known to alleviate or even cure a wide variety of ailments, including high blood pressure, arthritis, ulcers, tuberculosis, and heart disease. But, most of all, it helps us avoid disease by keeping our internal energies in a state of balance. When our energy becomes blocked or impeded, we get sick. Disease tells us that our energy flow needs to be adjusted. Tai chi helps us release the vitality locked within our tense, imbalanced bodies.

Many of us hope for a long life. But we want that life to be vigorous, healthy, and happy, even in old age. We also know that having a tranquil spirit plays a crucial role in helping us to endure our often troubled and troubling world. Given the pace of modern life, we can grow old very fast. Tai chi offers us a strategy for achieving not only calmness but also rejuvenation.

Chapter 1

guidelines
for your practice

A young man traveled to a foreign land to attend the school of
a famous teacher of Tao. When he arrived at the school he was
interviewed by the teacher.

"What do you wish from me?" the teacher asked.

"I wish to be your student and become the finest Taoist in all
the land," the young man replied. "How long must I study?"

"A minimum of twenty years," the teacher answered.

"Twenty years is a long time," said the young man. "What if I
studied twice as hard as all your other students?"

"Forty years," was the teacher's reply.

"Why is that?" the puzzled young man asked.

"When one is fixated on achievement, the mind becomes tight and
one is further from the Way than before," responded the teacher.

Where to Practice

Tai chi can be practiced in a variety of settings. In China, it is quite common to see people doing their morning tai chi routines in the park. Your yard or basement or living room might be a suitable spot, or perhaps a ball field or even a parking lot. You'll need at least a twelve-by-fifteen-foot space. It is best to minimize distractions from passersby, traffic, or noise. But as your concentration deepens, you will be better able to surmount such distracting elements.

When to Practice

It is important to respect the natural rhythms of the day. Being active in the morning and relaxing at night is the best way to nourish our spirits. A healthy schedule improves not only our tai chi practice but also our general health and well-being. It's worth the effort to establish a positive routine.

Many people find it convenient to practice tai chi in the morning, before breakfast and work. Some may even take the opportunity to practice again later in the day. Between 10 A.M. and 5 P.M. is an especially good time for exercise, because you are likely to have a half-empty stomach. (It is best not to practice tai chi for at least several hours after eating a meal.) Early birds may prefer a predawn or daybreak workout.

When ill with a cold or flu, you should just relax. Illness is a sign for us to rest. Take a break from physical exertion, including meditation or tai chi.

For people who do mental work, the best time to exercise is from 3 to 5 P.M. or about forty minutes before eating a light dinner. But don't forget that certain laws govern our bodies and minds. For example, if we spend a lot of time thinking in the evening, it is often difficult to stop thinking when we want to sleep. Similarly, undertaking physical movement just before retiring is not conducive to a restful night, and the abrupt change of pace can even damage our lungs and other organs.

When you exercise in the morning, start very slowly and gently. Energy is abundant in the early morning, but even then you must be moderate and avoid overstimulation.

And remember: everyone is different. Some people may make dramatic progress quickly. Others will improve at a slower rate. But each of us, if we are sincere, is capable of experiencing abiding change through the practice of tai chi.

How Much to Practice

Be moderate in your tai chi practice. Even a twenty-minute session is plenty. Usually it is best to do your practice deliberately, at a moderate pace. A routine done rapidly, especially before you are fully awake, may overstimulate you. But each person is unique, and our energy levels vary from day to day. Tailor your practice to your own rhythms. Observe how you feel. A fifteen- or twenty-minute session may feel sufficient, but you may find you want to practice again later in the day. It isn't necessary to complete the full eighteen-step routine: if you don't have the twenty minutes necessary to finish all the movements, you may opt to do only a portion of them. Respect your own internal clock. Become aware of your own tendencies. One day you might do just one of the eighteen movements, stop, and then do another. Another day you might choose to start in the middle of the eighteen and proceed from there.

When you exercise, stop before you are exhausted. A little tiredness is OK, such as when you climb stairs and get slightly out of breath. But do not overexert yourself. Build up your stamina gradually and gently. Stay relaxed. Tension is what hurts us, not serene, graceful movements.

Above all, do what you do for the pleasure it gives you. If you force yourself to do something, it will bring no benefit. But when you do it for enjoyment, you become a *shien*, or a person whose spirit is content.

Tai Chi and Diet

A light diet is best for practicing tai chi. Avoid too much bread or rice or other heavy carbohydrates. Serious tai chi students tend to eat very light foods such as Chinese porridge, which is a rice soup that is easily digested and therefore allows them to do tai chi again soon after eating. If you eat heavy foods until you are stuffed, you will need at least four hours to digest the meal. By the time you're able to do tai chi again, it will already be time for your next meal! Instead, eat light foods in small amounts.

Many of us enjoy splurging occasionally on gourmet foods. But don't let fine dining become an obstacle to your tai chi practice. You can indulge yourself on special occasions, but in general, moderation is best. And remember, whether you eat simple or gourmet food, do not practice tai chi on a full stomach.

Posture and the Spine

If your spine is poorly aligned, the qi that flows through it moves haltingly, to the detriment of your health. Correct posture is crucial in tai chi. The spine should always be aligned from the tailbone to the top of the neck, yet remain relaxed and flexible. You also should strive to keep your tailbone tucked forward, including the sphincter muscle around the anus. The chin should also be kept slightly tucked, and the head held erect, as if a string were attached to the crown of your head, pulling it up.

Good posture is a virtue to be cultivated at every moment of your life. Proper spinal alignment will enable your internal energy to flow unimpeded.

Center of Gravity

Our bodies have three regions called the three *tan tien* or "three origins." The upper *tan tien* is a point just above the top of the head and is regarded as the connecting point between the physical and the spiritual. The middle *tan tien* lies several inches below the throat and is associated with the heart or soul. The midpoint of the human body, just below the navel, is the lower *tan tien*. For men, the lower *tan tien* is the center of gravity in tai chi, the place from which their movements originate as they practice most exercises. Women, whose lower *tan tien* is already grounded, might choose to focus on the middle *tan tien* as the place from which their movements originate. The lower *tan tien* is connected to the energy of the earth, and keeping your center there strengthens your physical and sexual stamina.

Relax: Energy Is on the Way

Tai chi requires relaxed, attentive awareness. A muddled, distracted mind cannot give precise messages to the body. With a relaxed and uncluttered mind, the body can act with speed and precision. So rather than frantically pondering the world, worrying and analyzing, try to keep your mind free of extraneous thoughts and focused on the practice. The mental clarity that unfolds as we do our tai chi practice allows us to be "passively active": the mind will be both a neutral, relaxed observer and an active partner of the body and spirit.

The more focused you are during your tai chi practice, the more powerful its benefits will be. Your energy will evolve organically. You will begin to feel a sense of well-being not unlike the feeling that a warm spring breeze can evoke. Tai chi will help you nurture your true potential. As you deepen your connection to the truths of tai chi, your practice will become an enticing source of pleasure. The real secret to mastering tai chi is to enjoy yourself. As the ancient Taoist sage Lao Tzu emphasized, we don't achieve spiritual awareness through grim striving. So just relax, continue your practice, and let your spirit unfold naturally.

twelve principles of tai chi practice and daily life

Gracefulness of Body and Spirit

You can cultivate gracefulness by practicing tai chi, because it emphasizes balance, awareness, and a supple adaptation to the cadences of nature. Do all your movements in a gentle manner. Try not to thrash around. Relax. Moving qi through your body is a serene process. If you do anything abruptly, you might block the flow and end up with a headache or other ailment.

Evenness and Fullness

There is a special quality of tai chi called *zhong yun yuan mang*. *Zhong yun* means "evenness": nothing sticks out, nothing is unusual; even when you put special emphasis on a certain movement, an external observer will not notice it. *Yuan mang* means "fullness." To be full means that your whole body, from the *tan tien* at the base of your belly to your fingertips, from the soles of your feet to the top of your head, is full of energy. Combined, *zhong yun* and *yuan mang* refer to the energetic wholeness you will achieve as you practice.

Naturalness

Nothing about tai chi is superficial or artificial. Each of the movements describes a circle and is intrinsically related to the currents of energy that flow through our bodies. There are no abrupt changes in direction, speed, or style in tai chi. We just keep making circles: small ones, large ones, and horizontal, vertical, or slanted ones, in all directions. And all our movements are ultimately one movement, because they are all connected. Whether we reach out or gather in, the pattern is cyclical.

The ancient sages learned that we cannot resist our own natures. But no one needs to think about being natural. Even without the conscious mind, our bodies spontaneously seek a harmonious solution to any challenge. Practicing the ancient, soothing exercises of tai chi attunes us to the laws that govern both the flow of our internal energy and the flow of universal energy. As we become aware of the circular patterns in which energy moves through our bodies, we realize that our individual lives are small models of the universe.

The sages of old who discovered and developed the original energy-balancing exercises of tai chi hoped to maintain the natural wholeness of their spirits. Through tai chi movements they could imitate the stars that moved above them and activate the energies that swirled within them. And we can practice these same exercises today.

Simplicity

Our spirits thrive on simplicity. Sometimes it might seem that tai chi is rather complex, but it teaches us to manage this complexity in a direct, uncomplicated way. The simplicity we perfect through tai chi is a priceless tool in all our endeavors. Even the most complex structure, whether a business, a machine, or an idea, is best understood and mastered through simplicity. Simplicity is effective. When we complicate matters, we lose ourselves. Learn to be simple.

Gentleness

We must learn to be peaceful in speech, thought, emotion, and action. Wise people know that treating others violently is the same as treating ourselves violently. In tai chi, we learn to be gentle. To be direct and gentle in daily life is a manifestation of the truth that animates tai chi.

Flexibility

Reality constantly changes, challenging us to respond attentively. Since no situation is static, no prearranged response will do. Many people think life has to be a certain way; when life surprises them, they become nervous and want to assert control. However, when we are humble, without seeking to be in charge, we calmly permit life to flow.

Balance and Poise

Achieving balance and poise in movement is harder than we might think. For example, even when we are sitting still, are we actually calm and poised? As a matter of fact, many of us cannot even sit still. Through our practice of tai chi we learn grace and self-possession. We are able to handle challenging circumstances with newfound composure. It is important to find the equilibrium in our bodies that allows us to be balanced in stillness, even as we are in motion.

Calmness

Learn to be calm, especially in difficult situations. The flow of tai chi movement is calm. Most qi exercises follow this principle. Some styles of martial arts may be vigorous, but a violent force never lasts for long.

Kindness

Be kind to all beings. Tai chi is not damaging or harmful in any way.

Frugality

Both in daily life and in tai chi practice, we should protect our vital force and use it prudently. Do not be overly confident in your physical, material, and mental prowess, but be prepared. Practice restraint in your use of energy. Make sure you always have enough for any situation. If you are frugal with your energy, it will become abundant.

Yielding

Another principle of tai chi practice is to know the right time and place to use our energy. We must not squander our strength on foolishness. Tai chi movement never confronts force directly: it sidesteps it. The goal of yielding is not to give ground just for the sake of giving ground, but to triumph by avoiding confrontation.

Centeredness

Tai chi practice illustrates the principle of *zhong*, or centeredness. When we use our strength in tai chi practice, we must always be centered and able to keep our balance. Even a little too much exertion in one direction will be enough to make us fall over. To practice tai chi is to move smoothly and efficiently in a balanced stance.

Chapter 2

harmony tai chi
warm-up

*Warming up prior to starting tai chi is important,
because it activates the flow of qi in all parts of the
body and alleviates stress. The warm-up also may be
done by itself to promote energy circulation at any
time during the day.*

Awakening Qi in the Channels

These warm-up movements help to awaken or activate qi in the energy channels of the body.

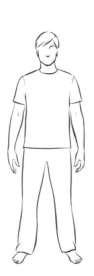 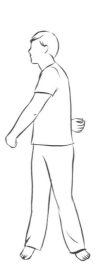 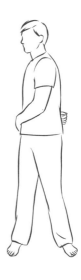

a. Tapping the trunk

Start with the feet shoulder-width apart. Let your arms hang down at your sides. Relax your body, especially the neck and shoulder muscles. Initiate a turning movement by shifting your weight from side to side, turning at the waist and pelvic area to cause your arms to swing. With loose fists, gently tap the area below your waist (slightly below the level of your navel) in front and back—the lower *tan tien*. The gentle weight shift or rocking from side to side will help give momentum to your arm swings.

BREATHING: Breathe deeply and naturally.

continued on next page

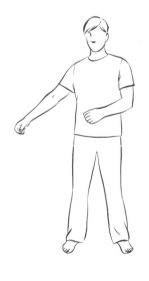
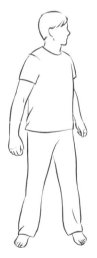
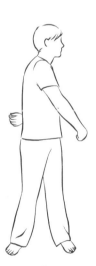
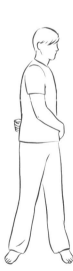

Gradually move the tapping motion up the center of your trunk and spine as high as you can comfortably reach and then back down to the lower *tan tien*. Repeat a few times.

BREATHING: Breathe deeply and naturally.

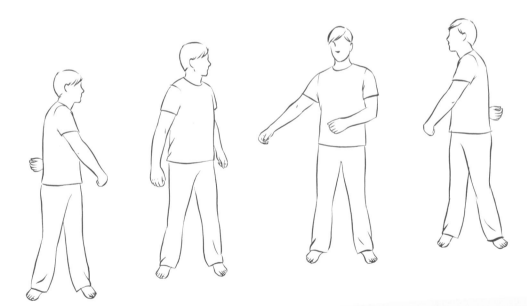

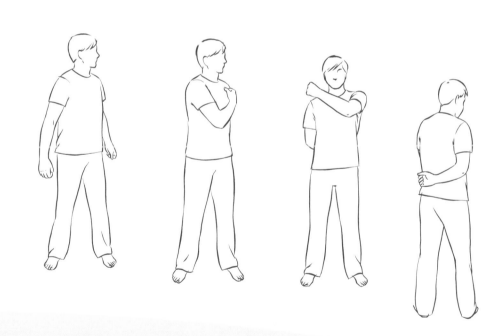

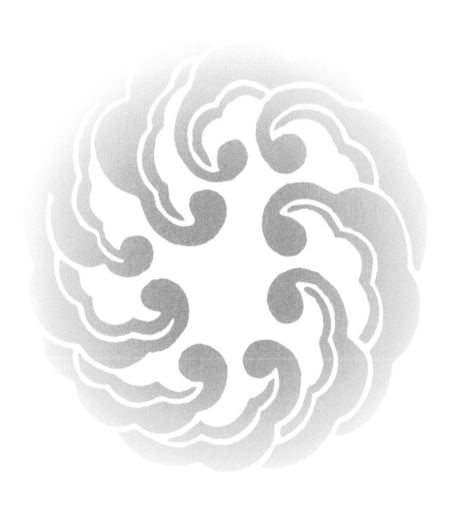

b. Tapping the trunk and arms

Start with the feet shoulder-width apart. Lift and extend the left arm out and slightly upward from the elbow. Make loose fists with both hands, and with the right fist tap from the level of the navel to under your left arm, up to the shoulder, and then up the inside of the left arm to the hand. Then turn your left arm so that your fist is pointing down, and tap back down the top side of the arm, beginning at the wrist, moving in along the shoulder to the neck.

BREATHING: Breathe deeply and naturally.

continued on next page

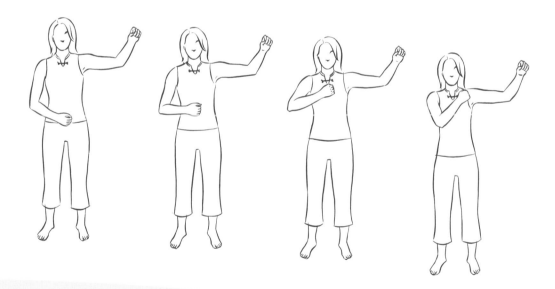

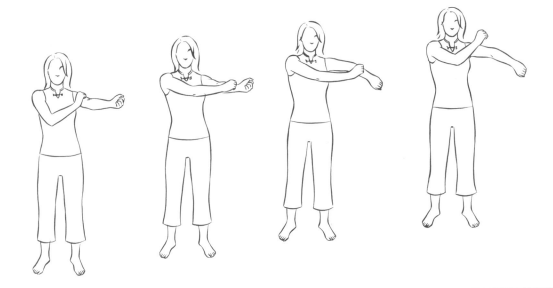

Repeat these motions on the other side with the right arm extended outward, tapping with the left hand in a loose fist.

continued on next page

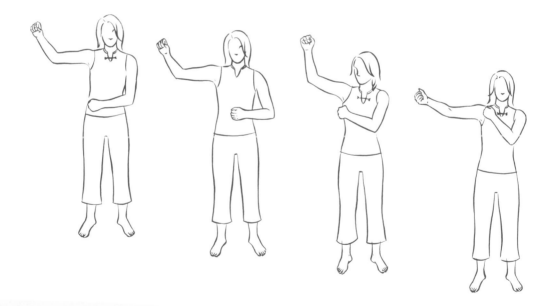

BREATHING: Breathe deeply and naturally.

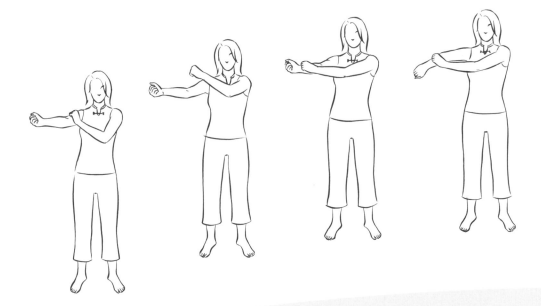

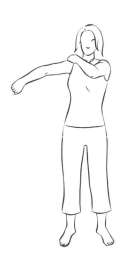

c. Tapping the trunk and legs

Start with the feet wide apart. Making loose fists with your hands, tap over the lower back; bend forward at the waist and continue tapping, out to the sides, down the sides of your legs (you can bend your knees to reach your ankles), and back in to the spine.

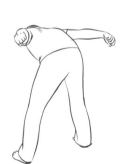 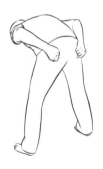 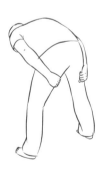 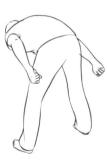

Still bending at the waist, continue tapping down along the sides of the buttocks and down the outside of the legs to the ankles (you can bend your knees to reach your ankles); then switch to the inside of the ankles as you tap up the inside of the legs to where the legs connect to the trunk (the ligaments on each side of the crotch).

BREATHING: Breathe deeply and naturally.

continued on next page

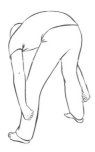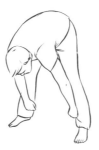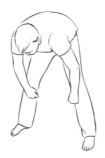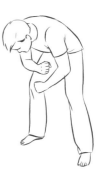

Come into a standing position.

Bring the feet in to shoulder-width apart and tap with the inside of your loose fists against the place where the legs connect to the trunk. Bend and straighten your knees a few times, creating an up and down motion while tapping.

BREATHING: Breathe deeply and naturally.

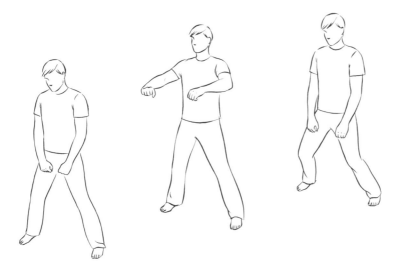

d. Swinging the arms back and jumping up

Start with the feet shoulder-width apart. Freely swing your arms back until you find the point of natural resistance, and then let them swing to the front again.

After several swings, to enhance the movement, bend your knees slightly as your arms swing backward and lift your heels as your arms swing forward.

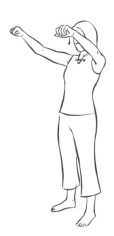 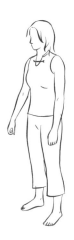 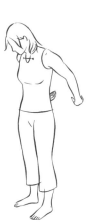 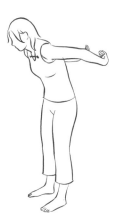

After several more swings, jump up as your arms swing forward. As you move your arms back and forth, feel as though the momentum of your arms swinging carries you up. Repeat, jumping progressively higher each time.

Then, gradually jump lower and lower. Slow down and gradually stop swinging your arms, bending your knees, and lifting your heels, and return to a normal standing position.

BREATHING: Inhale when your arms swing behind you.

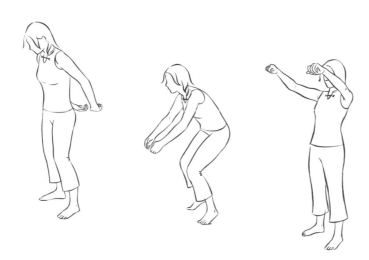

Loosening and Opening the Joints

These warm-up movements loosen and open the major joints of the body, allowing qi to pass through them more easily.

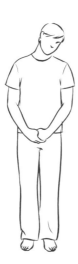 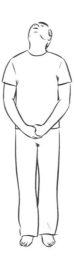 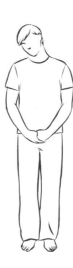

a. Circling the neck

Start with the heels together, feet turned out slightly and hands relaxed and clasped in front of abdomen.

Keeping the neck relaxed, allow gravity to roll the head forward. Gently and slowly roll your head to the left and then backward, making a wide circle. Repeat several times.

Reverse direction at a point when the head is bent forward, and repeat.

BREATHING: Inhale as your head circles to the back; exhale as it circles to the front.

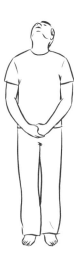 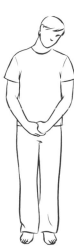

b. Turning the hips

Start with your feet together, or apart if necessary for balance. Place the palms of your hands over your kidneys and rub them a few times to warm them up.

Keep your palms over your kidneys. Hold your head upright and in line with your feet, and bend from the waist, as close to perpendicular to the ground as is comfortable, as you rotate your hips to the left, to the back, to the right, and forward to make a complete rotation. Repeat several times.

Reverse direction and repeat several more times, then straighten up.

BREATHING: Exhale as your hips circle forward; inhale as they circle back.

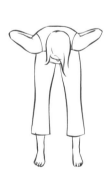 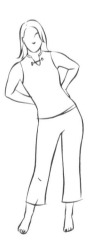 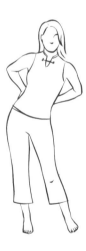

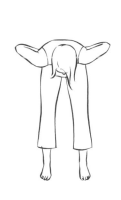 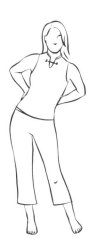 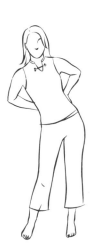

c. Turning the knees

Start with your feet together. Bend forward at the waist and rest your hands on your knees. Keep your knees together. Bend your knees as deeply as is comfortable, and lightly rub the knees to warm them. Make a smooth circling motion by rotating your bent knees clockwise around to the right, straightening them in mid-rotation, and coming back around to the front. You are creating a circle on a vertical axis, in which you start low, are higher in mid-rotation, and come back around to the lower starting point. Repeat several times. Reverse direction and circle several more times.

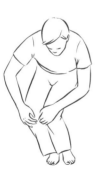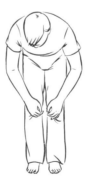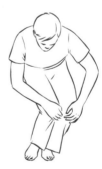

BREATHING: Exhale when bending your knees; inhale when straightening them.

continued on next page

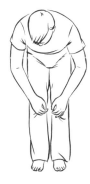 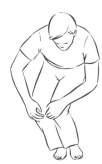

Next, begin with your knees straightened. Keeping your feet together, bend your knees forward and gently push them apart, circling them around to come back together; straighten up as your knees meet. Again, you are making a circle on a vertical axis—low when you are bending your knees, and gradually higher as you circle around to straighten them. Repeat several more times. Reverse the direction of the circles and repeat.

BREATHING: Exhale when bending your knees; inhale when straightening them.

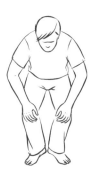 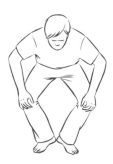 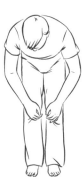

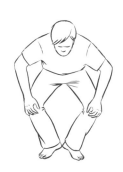

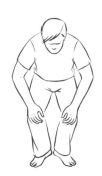

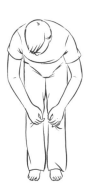

d. Turning the ankles

Begin with your hands on your hips. Lift the left foot. Rotate it at the ankle several times in one direction, then in the other. Alternate pointing and flexing the foot, then shake it to loosen the ankle joint. Repeat for the other foot.

NOTE: If you are having trouble balancing, you can steady yourself by resting a hand on the wall or another surface until you feel comfortable balancing on your own.

BREATHING: Breathe deeply and naturally.

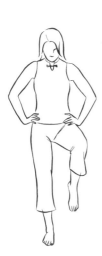
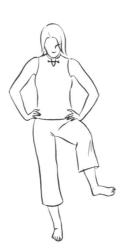
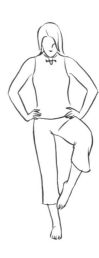

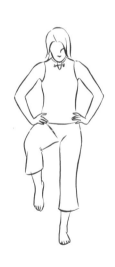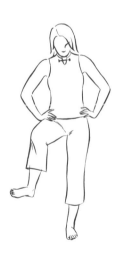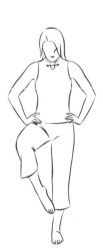

Chapter 3

harmony tai chi basic stances

There are six basic stances in Harmony Tai Chi that the beginner should learn: the Horse stance, the Cat stance, the Heel stance, the Bow (or Front) stance, the Twist stance, and the Half-Step.

Basic Positioning Guidelines

DIAGONAL POSITIONS

Throughout the descriptions of the tai chi movements, you will see references to positioning yourself on a diagonal. This refers to the position in which you are standing. You begin the series of movements facing front, but as you move though the movements, you will change the direction you face, turning on diagonals in 45-degree increments. When beginning to practice these tai chi movements, take note of what is in front of you. Perhaps it is a plant or a window; whatever it is, this is your **front**. If you move 90 degrees to your **right**, you will now be facing squarely right. Facing front again, if you turn 90 degrees to your **left**, you will be facing squarely left. And if from front you turn 180 degrees, you will now be facing your **rear**.

Positioning yourself diagonally, which you'll see often in the directions, is to position yourself facing 45 degrees from your front or rear. The diagonals are the four directions you face when you are in between front, right, rear, and left. Take a look at the Diagonals Diagram and you will see that the figure is facing front. If the figure turns 45 degrees to his right, he is now on the **right front diagonal**. If the figure turns from his front 45 degrees to his left, he is on a **left front diagonal**. If he continues to turn to his left, at the next 45-degree turn he will be facing left, and at the next 45-degree turn from there, he will now be facing the **left rear diagonal**, in between the left and the rear. Of course it would follow that if the figure turned 90 degrees from his front to his right, and then 45 more degrees toward the rear, he would be on the **right rear diagonal**, in between the right and the rear.

To apply this directional positioning in your tai chi practice, you simply stand in whatever stance you are supposed to be in, only your torso is turned to whatever direction is suggested. For example, if you are in Cat stance on the right front diagonal, your front foot is still pointed straight ahead, but "ahead" in this case means 45 degrees to the right from your front. These directional prompts are here to help guide you through the turning that occurs in Tai Chi movement.

DIAGONALS DIAGRAM

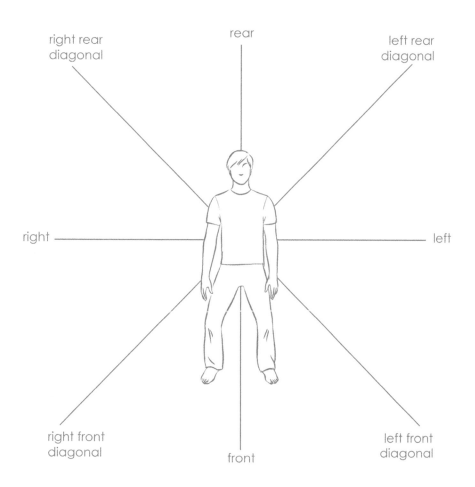

right rear
diagonal

rear

left rear
diagonal

right

left

right front
diagonal

front

left front
diagonal

WEIGHT PLACEMENT

In the movement instructions, you will see directions telling you to put varying percentages of your weight on one foot. Before beginning, practice getting accustomed to approximating your weight distribution. Following are general guidelines. Don't worry too much about the precise percentages, just focus on keeping your balance as you practice these movements.

90 percent / 10 percent: This means that you should put all of your weight on one foot, then press very slightly on the opposite foot until you feel it balancing the pose only, and not supporting any substantial amount of weight. You should feel the muscles in the 90 percent leg really activating here.

80 percent / 20 percent: Begin in 90/10 and then bend the 10 percent leg, adding a nominal amount of weight to the gentle balance. Your 90 percent leg should feel a small degree of relief in the activating muscles as 10 percent of the weight is transferred. You will feel a very gentle activation of the muscles in the 20 percent leg.

70 percent / 30 percent: Begin with your weight evenly distributed on both legs. Now shift a little of the weight from one leg to the other, until you feel a slight sense of one leg being slightly longer; this is the 30 percent leg. Both legs are supporting the weight, but the muscles are activated more in the 70 percent leg, which will be slightly bent.

60 percent / 40 percent: From the 70/30, shift a little bit more of your weight from the 70 percent leg and feel the slight relief as you disengage the muscles on this leg slightly. Here there is a very subtle difference between the weight on each leg, but the 60 percent leg is still working harder.

50 percent / 50 percent: You feel equal weight on both legs.

Now practice moving from 90/10 to 80/20 to 70/30 to 60/40 to 50/50 and back again until you feel comfortable that you can feel the differences.

Basic Stances

The following descriptions will give you an idea of the positions you will be in during each of the stances. When they are combined into different tai chi movements, you might form the stances differently from the way they are described here, and your hands and arms may be in different positions. For example, you may step forward rather than backward to form a stance, and your hands may be raised.

1. The Horse Stance

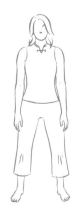

Stand with your feet pointing straight ahead, shoulder-width apart, with your knees slightly bent, waist loose, and shoulders relaxed. Your weight should be evenly distributed across both feet, your arms hanging naturally at your sides.

2. The Cat Stance

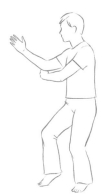

With your feet pointing straight ahead, shoulder-width apart, step one foot back, turned out at a forty-five-degree angle. Raise the heel of the front foot so that you are balancing (that is, very gently resting) 10 percent of your weight on the ball of your foot, and shift 90 percent (that is, almost all) of your weight to the rear foot. Keep your knees slightly bent and your trunk facing the same direction as your front foot. The arm on the same side as the front foot should be held gently aloft and bent at the elbow, while the arm on the side of your rear foot should be held gently in front of your torso, also bent at the elbow with your hand in a fist. If it is less confusing, your arms can hang naturally at your sides for now.

3. The Heel Stance

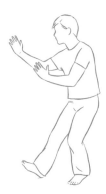

With your feet pointing straight ahead, shoulder-width apart, step one foot back, turned out at a forty-five-degree angle. Raise the ball of the front foot to balance 10 percent of your body weight on the heel and shift 90 percent of your weight to the rear foot. Keep your knees slightly bent and your trunk facing the same direction as your front foot. As in the Cat stance, the arm on the same side as the front foot should be held gently aloft and bent at the elbow, while the arm on the side of your rear foot should be held gently in front of your torso, also bent at the elbow. Again, if it is less confusing for now, your arms can hang naturally at your sides.

4. The Bow (or Front) Stance

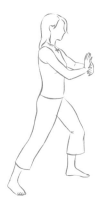

With your feet pointing straight ahead, wide apart, take a big step back with one foot, turning it out at a forty-five-degree angle. Bend the knee of the front leg, and keep the knee of the rear leg almost straight. Your front foot should be bearing 70 percent of your weight, with your back foot helping to support and balance you by carrying 30 percent of your weight. Make sure your heels are not in the same line. Your trunk should face the same direction as your front foot, and your arms should be poised horizontally with bent elbows in front of your torso, with the hand that is on the same side as the front foot curled around the other hand. If you prefer, you can let your arms hang naturally at your sides for now.

5. The Twist Stance

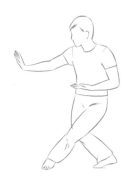

This transition step often occurs after a Cat stance. In that case, lift the lead foot, move it forward a little, and touch the ground heel first; as you place the rest of the front foot down, turn it outward. As you transfer your weight forward to the front foot by bending your knee, your torso should gently turn until it faces the same direction as the pointed leading foot. Lift the heel of your rear foot, bending the knee gently, so you are resting on the ball of that foot. When you feel comfortable with this movement, add the arms: the lead arm moves back until the elbow tucks like a folded wing with the palm facing up, while the rear arm smoothly pushes forward.

6. The Half-Step

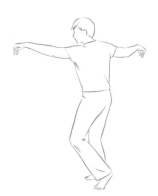

The Half-Step often comes after the Twist stance and before another stance, such as the Bow stance. When learning the pose, start with your feet together. Shift 80 percent of your weight onto one foot as you raise the heel of the other. Your arms come out, spreading apart like wings, with the arm on the side of the 20 percent foot reaching forward and the other reaching backward, your elbows slightly bent and your fingers gently dangling. (If you come from the Twist stance, you would move your rear leg forward in line with your front foot and shift 80 percent of your weight onto that leg as you switch your arms by pushing forward the arm that was once back, and pulling back the arm that was once forward.)

Chapter 4

harmony tai chi short form

Important Points to Remember
before Doing Eighteen-Step Harmony Tai Chi

1. Relax! This is perhaps the most important principle in tai chi. Most of us tend to hold tension in various parts of our bodies, such as the shoulders and lower back. As you proceed through the tai chi movements, check your entire body for tension. Wherever you find tension, relax and release it. That will help you move more smoothly and freely. In fact, this is a valuable general principle for every endeavor in life.

2. Move your whole body as a single unit. No part of your body should move in isolation from the whole. All movements should be integrated and connected.

3. All moves originate in your feet, find direction in your waist, and are expressed by your arms and hands. Think of the movements as waves rippling through your body.

4. Be solid and rooted in your feet and light in your arms and head. Keep your head centered over your pelvis, meaning that if you were to draw a straight line from your pelvis to your head, they would always be aligned with each other on the same vertical axis.

5. Expand your back and relax your chest inward slightly. Instead of keeping your body erect and taut, which does not facilitate practicing smooth and gentle motions, keep your back slightly curled. You are engaging your muscles, but not tensing them to remain erect, and you are also gently poised to move smoothly from one movement to the next.

6. Move slowly and naturally. This will allow you to check carefully for any incorrect or unbalanced movements. Gradually cultivate stability and fluidity.

7. Your mind should be quiet and focused. That will help direct your energy while you are proceeding through the movements. Do not think of the motion as using muscular force, but rather as naturally rolling through the movements, using fluid energy.

8. When you are first learning a movement, don't worry about coordinating your breathing with the movement. Just breathe naturally. Breathe deeply from your diaphragm, keeping your lower abdomen relaxed.

   Once you have learned the movements, you can try to coordinate them with your breathing, but don't be rigid. In general, as your hands rise or pull back toward the body, breathe in; as your hands descend or push away from the body, breathe out.

9. The tip of your tongue should lightly touch your upper palate. When the tongue is positioned this way, it is nearly impossible to clench your jaw. This soft detail will promote an overall feeling of peace in all your movements.

10. Relax your shoulders and have a slight bend in your elbows.

11. Relax your lower back and tuck your pelvis under slightly.

eighteen-step harmony tai chi

movement 0:
The Great Void

Common Tai Chi Name: Wu Chi

The opening stance is called "the Great Void" and symbolizes the unmanifested energy (creative stillness, primal female or mysterious "mother" aspect) of the Tao. Stand in a Horse stance, facing forward with your knees slightly bent, your waist and shoulders relaxed, your chin tucked in slightly, your hands at your sides, your pelvis tucked under as if you were getting ready to sit down, and your mind clear. Curl your tongue so that the tip is lightly touching the roof of your mouth.

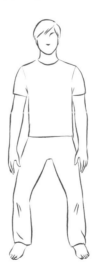

movement 1:
Existence before Heaven and Earth

Common Tai Chi Name: Beginning Tai Chi
This is the first movement of the Harmony Tai Chi form. Its general purpose is to activate the main energy centers of the body (the lower, middle, and upper *tan tien*), connecting them to one another and to the environment.

a. While in the Horse stance facing forward, slowly raise both hands waist high, palms down, bending your elbows to waist level (slightly above lower *tan tien*).

b. Slowly return your hands to your sides.

c. Raise both hands slowly to eyebrow level (above the middle *tan tien*), palms facing down.

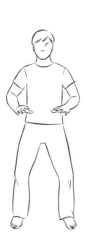

a.

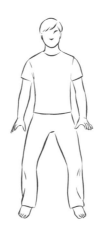

b.

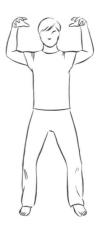

c.

d. Bring your hands, palms still facing down, downward toward the middle *tan tien* (heart) level and push them straight out with your palms facing forward. Do not lock your elbows when extending your arms.

e. Bring your hands back toward your body and up toward the top of your head (above the upper *tan tien*). Keep your palms facing forward with the fingers pointing to the sky. Stop when your hands are about six inches in front of your head.

f. Let your hands descend slowly to your sides.

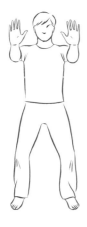

d.

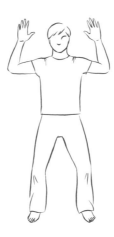

e.

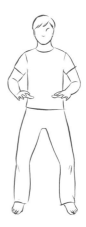

f.

movement 2:
Gate of Subtle Origin

Common Tai Chi Name: Grasp the Sparrow's Tail
This movement is actually a sequence of five different movements, which are explained below. You first perform a transition movement followed by the following four movements: Raise the Lower (a.k.a. Brush Sleeve or Ward Off), Lower the Elevated (or, Roll Back), Decrease the Overabundant (or, Press), and Nourish the Insufficient (or, Push).

1. Mini Cloud Hands Transition

a. While in the Horse stance, turn your torso to face the right front diagonal direction and circle your right hand clockwise up across the body to shoulder level with palm down (your elbow should be lower than your wrist), while at the same time turning your left hand palm up and bringing it to the lower *tan tien*. Both hands should now be positioned as if holding a "ball" of energy. As you move, gently bend into your knee as you shift 60 percent of your weight to the right foot.

a.

b. Turn your body to face the left front diagonal direction as you circle the left hand outward and up toward the left to shoulder level with palm down (your elbow should be lower than your wrist), while at the same time turning your right hand palm up and bringing it to the lower *tan tien*. As you move, gently bend into your knee as you shift 60 percent of your weight to the left foot.

c. Rotate your left foot outward (pivot on the heel) to the left front diagonal. Then shift all of your weight to the left foot as you bring the ball of your right foot next to the left heel to form a Half-Step stance. Your arms have not moved, but are still holding the ball of energy.

continued on next page

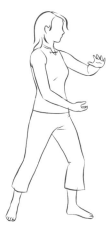

b.

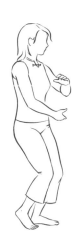

c.

2. Raise the Lower

Common Tai Chi Name: Brush Sleeve or Ward Off

d. Step out with your right foot to form a right Bow stance on the right front diagonal.

Rotate your left foot toward the front at a forty-five-degree angle (pivot on the heel), bring your right arm under your left arm with palm up, and brush the left sleeve, moving the right palm past the left elbow, left forearm, and left wrist. Bring the right arm forward and outward to chest level with your palm facing your body while bringing your left hand down toward your left hip with your palm down and parallel to the ground.

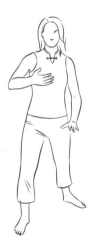

d.

3. Lower the Elevated

Common Tai Chi Name: Roll Back

e. From the previous position, circle your left hand out and to the front, palm up, to the same level as your right hand, which is still at chest level. And raise your right arm to shoulder level while turning your right palm up.

f. Then turn both hands palms down, rotate your left foot outward toward a left front diagonal as you swing both arms down and to the left, and shift your weight to your left foot while rotating your right foot (pivoting on heel) to the left front diagonal.

g. At the end of the arm swing, your left palm and elbow should be facing left, at waist level. Your right palm is beginning to face up near the lower *tan tien*. Raise your arm until it reaches chest level. Your weight should be on the left foot, and the right foot should be rotated to face the left front diagonal.

continued on next page

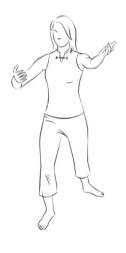

e.

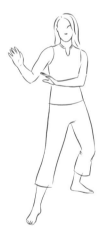

f.

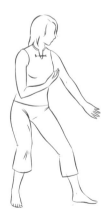

g.

h. Shift your weight backward to your right foot and bring your left heel up to form a Cat stance facing left. The left palm and elbow should still be facing out to the left. As you continue through these movements, momentarily twist your torso to the right front diagonal and back again.

i. Bring your left arm upward, toward the chest, turning your palm gradually inward as you gently bend your elbow to reach the middle *tan tien*. (As you do this, do not raise your left shoulder.) At the same time, bring the right hand to the middle *tan tien*, above the left, and rest the base of the right palm on top of the left wrist.

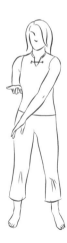

h.

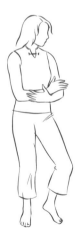

i.

4. Decrease the Overabundant

Common Tai Chi Name: Press

j. Still in the Cat Stance, you have shifted your body back to a left diagonal. Keep your hands together and press your arms forward as you step out with your left foot and transfer your weight to this foot to form a Bow stance facing left. The left arm should be horizontal to the ground, palm facing torso. The base of the right palm should press against the left wrist and rest on top of it as your arms push forward together. The hands should not extend beyond the front knee, which means your elbows are bent.

continued on next page

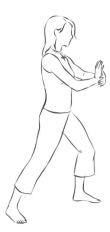

j.

5. Nourish the Insufficient

Common Tai Chi Name: Push

k.   From the previous stance, transfer your weight to the rear foot and come into a left Cat stance, meaning that 10 percent of your weight is on the ball of your left foot. Circle your right arm up just above your left elbow.

l.   With your right palm brush the left arm from the elbow to the back of the left hand; your left hand, meanwhile, is moving down to your lower *tan tien*. The whole right hand should extend over the left arm in this brushing motion.

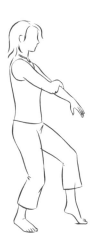

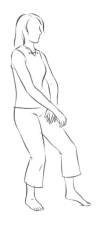

l.

k.

m. Circle both hands, palms facing down, up and back toward the upper *tan tien* (forehead), till they are about six inches in front of your head; then gently push the hands down through the middle *tan tien* (heart level) to the lower *tan tien* (waist level).

n. Step your left leg forward into a Bow stance facing left, and at the same time push both hands forward, palms facing outward, from the lower *tan tien* in an upward semi-arc to chest level. Hands should not extend beyond the front knee.

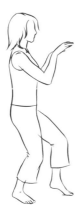

m.

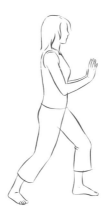

n.

movement 3:
Exposition of the Heavenly Mystery (Yang within Yin)

Common Tai Chi Name: Double Whip
This movement consists of two circling arms. The right arm moves in a larger circle above as the left arm moves in a smaller circle below. The left represents the yang energy and the right represents the yin.

a. From the left Bow stance, shift your weight onto the rear right leg as you rotate to the right (pivot on the right and left heels) and turn your feet to the front. At the same time, circle your body and arms toward the front, turning the left palm upward and the right palm downward, both at chest level.

b. When the arms have reached the front, shift your weight to the left leg and bring the right foot next to the left heel to form a Half-Step stance facing front. At the same time, pivot your wrists to form a crane's beak with the left hand (all five fingers touching and facing downward) and bring your right palm (fingers facing upward) to press outward against the inside of the beak.

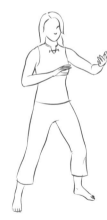

a.

b.

c. Scoop the right hand down and backward toward the left armpit, and then rest it, palm up, atop the bicep of the left arm, which is starting to drop slightly.

d. Circle the right hand horizontally outward and clockwise, palm up, brushing atop the left arm. Keep the right elbow slightly bent. At the same time, open the left hand, turn it from palm down to palm forward, and circle it clockwise until it is under the right armpit. While the arms circle, turn the right foot to the right, set it flat on the ground, and transfer your weight onto it. Raise up the left heel and rotate on the ball of the foot so that the left foot is now aligned with the right front diagonal.

e. At full extension of this circling motion, both palms should face upward, the left palm below the right armpit. The right arm, barely bent, extends out to the right. The arms should circle as far as the right rear diagonal.

continued on next page

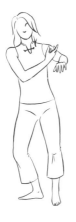

c.

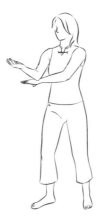

d.

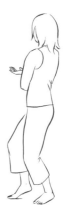

e.

f. Bring the right arm in toward the chest with the palm facing left; as you do this, pull the left hand through the right armpit, turn it palm downward, and bring it toward your right wrist. At the same time, shift your weight to the rear leg to form a Cat stance facing the right. The hands should meet at the middle *tan tien* (in front of the heart), with the left palm edge resting on the back of the right wrist. The right palm should be vertical and facing the left front diagonal.

g. With the hands in this position, step forward with the right leg making a Heel stance. Transition to Bow stance facing right.

h. Push the joined hands against one another and also slightly forward while at the same time pushing your torso forward. The joined hands should not extend beyond the front knee, and the right palm should still be facing the left front diagonal.

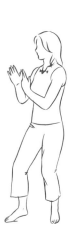

f.

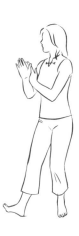

g.

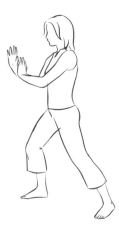

h.

movement 4:

Empty, Yet Productive

Common Tai Chi Name: Brush Knee, Left Side

A transitional twisting stance precedes this actual movement. Then, the left hand circles twice, first vertically in the direction of the body, then horizontally toward the outside of the left knee.

a. From the right Bow stance, shift your weight to the rear leg to form a Cat stance facing right. At the same time, let the arms descend to hip level, separate your hands, and raise them to shoulder level, palms down, and extend them in opposite directions. Right arm should be forward, left arm backward. Elbows should be slightly bent when arms are extended.

b. Step out with the right foot to form a Twist stance. Transfer your weight to the right leg. As your weight is slowly transferred to the right leg, turn the right palm up and bring your right elbow in toward the right side of your torso. At the same time, bend the left elbow toward the left side of your torso and bring the left palm forward, face down, toward the right palm.

continued on next page

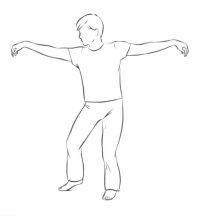

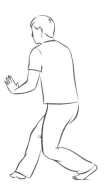

a.

b.

c. Brush the left palm (palm down) clockwise just above the right palm (palm up) and extend the left arm out to the left side. The curved right arm is gently being drawn back, into the torso, and then brushes by on the right side until your right arm is pointing straight out to the right. At the same time, raise the left heel slightly, as you twist more to the right.

Step up with the left foot to form a Half-Step stance, with 80 percent of your weight remaining on the right foot. Continue to circle your right arm slowly around until it is straight out to the right at head level. Simultaneously, widely circle your straightened left arm upward and around from your side to just in front of your face until you are looking at the inside of your palm.

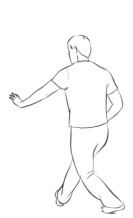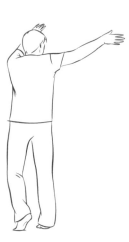

c.

d. With your left palm still facing your torso, continue to move your left arm around in its wide circle to the right. Briefly float your arm just beyond the right armpit then circle it down, turning your palm down as you do, to the level of the lower *tan tien*, and ending a foot above your left thigh. The right arm is straight out to the right at head level; bend your elbow and push your hand, palm down, to just beside your right ear.

e. Put all of your weight on your right leg momentarily as you step out with the left leg into a left Bow stance. Pivot on your right flat foot until it's on a forty-five-degree angle. Your left hand continues to float palm down, now about six inches above your knee. Meanwhile, you extend the right hand forward, past the ear, at shoulder level, palm turning up to face forward, elbow slightly bent. The right hand should not extend beyond the left knee.

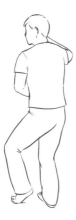

d.

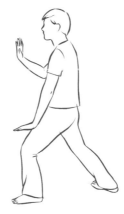

e.

movement 5:
The Greatly Skilled Seems Clumsy

Common Tai Chi Name: Playing the Lute, Left Side
In this movement, both arms circle down to gather from below, as if scooping energy from the earth. The left hand ends up in front of the right as if you're playing a harp.

a. Rock more of your weight onto the left foot and lift the right heel while moving your torso forward.

b. Take a tiny step forward with your right foot and shift 90 percent of your weight back to the right foot, to transition into a Cat stance facing left. Bring the left arm up, with elbow bent, and turn it horizontal to the ground, and turn the right forearm down toward the left, also horizontal to the ground, so that your forearms overlap horizontally, with the right arm above the left. Arms should be at shoulder level.

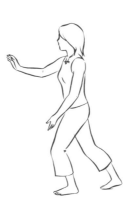

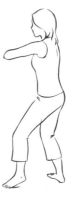

b.

a.

c. Lower your left heel to the floor and shift your weight so that it is distributed evenly on your flat feet, with your left foot still slightly forward. Straighten arms horizontally outward and then circle them downward (as if scooping up energy from the earth). During downward circling, bend the knees while keeping the back straight (not curved) and leaning forward slightly. As you circle your hands around, with palms up, they should cross at the wrists with the right hand over the left. Straighten your knees.

d. Uncross your wrists and raise your arms up the center of your torso with the left arm in front (bent at a forty-five-degree angle), palm facing right, and the right open hand near the left elbow, facing the elbow. At the same time, lift up the left front foot, transitioning briefly into a left-facing Cat stance with 10 percent of your weight on the ball, and then raise the ball of the foot to form a Heel stance facing the left.

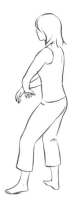

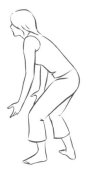

c.

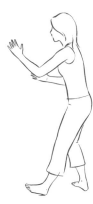

d.

movement 6:
Empty, Yet Productive

Common Tai Chi Name: Brush Knee, Ride Side
This movement is preceded by a transitional twisting stance—a mirror image of what you did in movement 4.

a. From the left Heel stance, let the arms descend to hip level and then raise them to shoulder level, palms down, so that they are extended in opposite directions. Your left arm should be forward, right arm backward. Elbows should be slightly bent when arms are extended, and palms should face down. At the same time, raise your left heel.

b. Step out with the left foot to form a Twist stance. Transfer your weight to the right leg. As weight is slowly transferred to the right leg, turn the left palm up and bring your left elbow in toward your torso. At the same time, bend the right elbow toward the right side of your torso and bring the right palm forward, face down, toward the left palm.

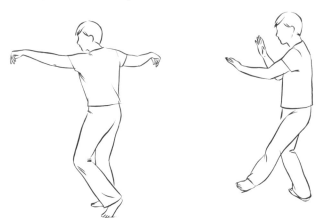

a.

b.

c. Brush the right palm (turned down) just above the left palm (palm up) and extend the right arm out to the right side. The curved left arm is gently drawing back into the left side of the torso. At the same time, raise the right heel, as you twist more to the left.

d. Step up with the right foot to form a Half-Step stance (weight should remain on the left leg). Continue to circle the left arm slowly around until it is straight out to the left at head level, palm up. Simultaneously, widely circle the straightened right arm upward and around from your side at head level to just in front of your face until you are looking at the inside of your right palm. The right arm continues to move around in its wide circle to the left, briefly floating just beyond the left armpit, circling down (the palm turning down) to the level of the lower *tan tien*, and ending about a foot above your left thigh. The left arm is straight out to the left at head level; bend your elbow and push your hand, palm down, to just beside your left ear.

continued on next page

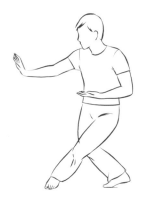

c.

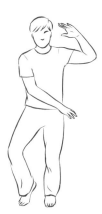

d.

e. Put all of your weight on your left leg momentarily as you step forward with the right leg into a right Bow stance. Pivot on your left flat foot until it's on a forty-five-degree angle. Your right hand continues to float palm down, now about six inches above your right knee. Meanwhile, the left hand extends forward, past the ear, at shoulder level, palm turning up to face forward, elbow slightly bent. The left hand should not extend beyond the right knee.

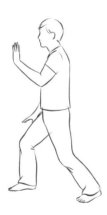

e.

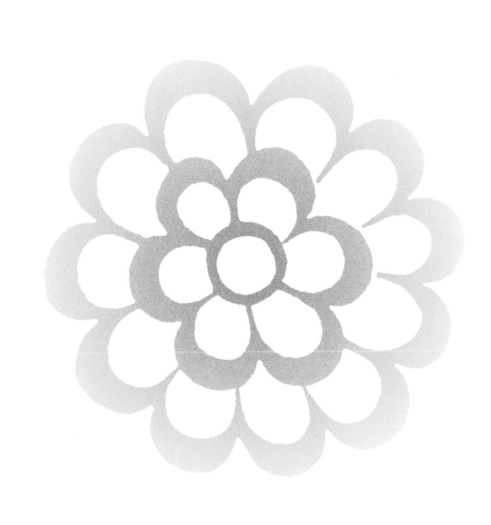

movement 7:
The Greatly Skilled Seems Clumsy

Common Tai Chi Name: Playing the Lute, Right Side
This movement is simply a mirror image of the instructions you followed in movement 5.

a. Rock more of your weight onto the right foot and lift the left heel while moving your torso forward.

b. Take a tiny step forward with your left foot and shift 90 percent of your weight back to the left foot, to transition into a Heel stance facing right with the ball of right foot slightly raised. Bring the right forearm up, with elbow bent, and turn it horizontal to the ground, and move the left forearm down toward the right, also horizontal to the ground, so that they overlap horizontally with the right arm over the left. Arms should be at shoulder level.

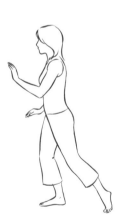

a.

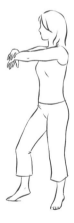

b.

c. Lower your right heel to the floor and shift your weight so that it is distributed evenly on your flat feet, with your right foot still slightly forward. Straighten arms horizontally outward and then circle them downward (as if scooping up energy from the earth).

d. During downward circling, bend the knees while keeping the back straight (not curved) and leaning forward slightly. As you circle your arms around, the hands, with palms up, should cross at the wrists with the left hand over the right. Begin to straighten your knees.

e. Uncross your wrists and raise your arms up the center of your torso with the right arm in front (bent at a forty-five-degree angle), palm facing left, and the left open hand near the right elbow, facing the elbow. At the same time, lift up the right front foot, transitioning briefly into a right-facing Cat Stance with 10 percent of your weight on the ball, and then set it down to form a Heel stance facing the right.

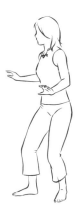

c.

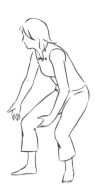

d.

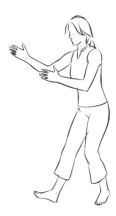

e.

movement 8:
To Be Curled Is to Be Straight

Common Tai Chi Name: Fist under Elbow
This movement starts with the arms curled and ends with them straightened—
again demonstrating an interplay of the opposite expression of yin and yang.

a. From the Heel stance, lift your right hand and elbow slightly. At the same
time, form a vertical fist with your left hand and place it briefly under the
right elbow, while lifting the front foot and setting it down to form a Cat
stance facing right.

b. Step forward with your right foot, plant it flat, and put your weight on it as
you bring your left fist forward from under your right elbow to begin a gentle
left punch as your right arm starts to recede behind you.

c. As you complete your left punch, bring your left foot into a Horse stance
and swing your right arm backward so it extends behind you.

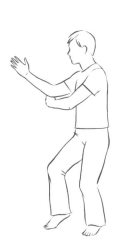

a.

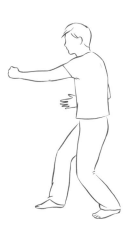

b.

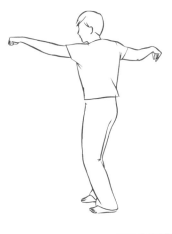

c.

movement 9:

To Progress in Tao Seems like Regressing

Common Tai Chi Name: Repulse the Monkey
This movement is an interplay of hands coming together and moving away. Each hand takes a turn at pushing off the palm of the other. The first three movements in this sequence will be stationary with three repetitions of arm extentions.

a. Now open the left fist and, keeping both arms extended, turn your hands palms down. Turn the body at the waist slightly to the right.

b. Then turn the palms upward and bring the right hand forward so it brushes past the right ear, while drawing the left hand back toward the body at chest level. At the same time, turn the body at the waist to face forward.

c. Continue to draw the left arm back, and the right arm forward, and brush the right palm over the left palm.

continued on next page

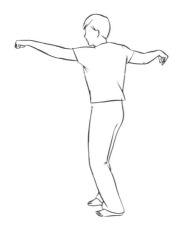

a.

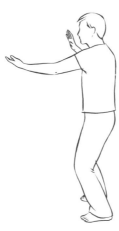

b.

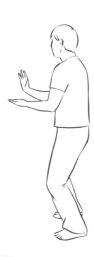

c.

d. Extend the right arm forward while moving the left arm down toward the waist (palm up).

e. Extend the left arm behind you (palm down). At full extension, both palms should be face down, your body turned at the waist slightly to the left.

f. Then circle the left hand forward so it brushes past the left ear (palm forward), while drawing the right hand, palm up, back toward the body at chest level. At the same time, turn the body at the waist to face forward.

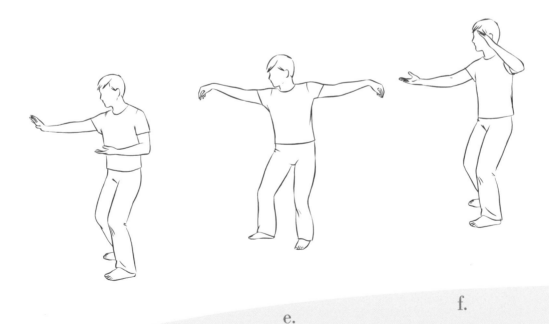

d.

e.

f.

g. Continue to draw the right arm back, and the left arm forward, and brush the left palm over the right palm. The body continues to turn toward the right at the waist.

h. Extend the left arm forward while moving the right arm down toward the waist (palm up).

i. Extend the right arm behind you (palm down). At full extension, both palms should be face down, your body turned at the waist slightly to the right.

continued on next page

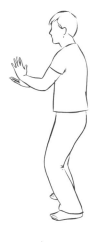
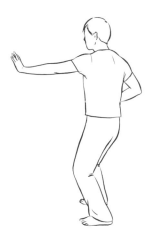
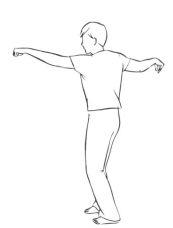

g.

h.

i.

j. From the previous position, shift your weight onto the right foot and bring your left foot next to the right heel to form a Half-Step stance.

k. Step back with your left leg (touching the ground toe first), turn the left palm up, and begin bringing your right palm forward, palm still face down, to brush past the right ear.

l. Transfer your weight to the left foot to form a Cat stance facing right. At the same time, turn the body to the left, bring your left arm back toward the body at chest level, and brush your right palm forward past the left palm.

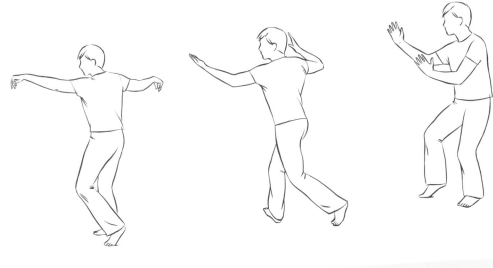

j.

k.

l.

m. Extend your right hand past the left palm. The right palm should face forward. The left palm should be up.

n. Withdraw your left arm to the rear. Extend both arms with palms down. Elbows should not be locked.

o. Step back with your right leg (resting on the ball of your right foot), turn the right palm up, and begin bringing your left palm forward, to brush past the left ear.

continued on next page

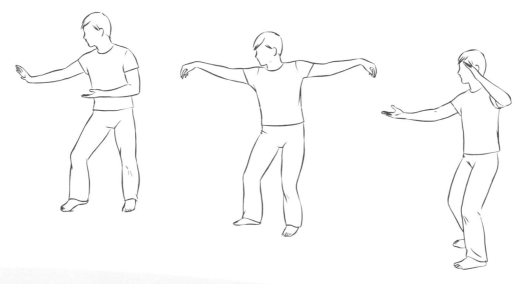

m.

n.

o.

p. Transfer your weight to the right foot to form a Cat stance facing left. At the same time, turn the body to the right, bring your right arm back toward the body at chest level, and brush your left palm forward past the right palm.

q. Extend your left hand past the right palm. The left palm should face forward. The right palm should be face up.

r. Withdraw your right arm to the rear. Extend both arms with palms down. Elbows should not be locked.

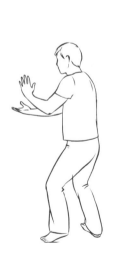

p.

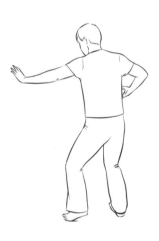

q.

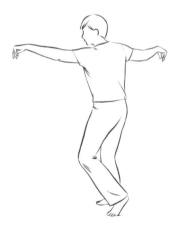

r.

s. Step back with your left leg (resting on the ball of your left foot), turn the left palm up, and begin bringing your right palm forward, to brush past the right ear.

t. Transfer your weight to the left foot to form a Cat stance facing right. At the same time, turn the body to the left, bring your left arm back toward the body at chest level, and brush your right palm forward past the left palm.

u. Extend your right hand past the left palm. The right palm should face forward. The left palm should face up, next to the waist.

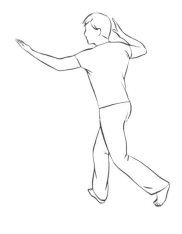

s.

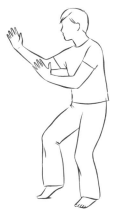

t.

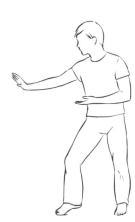

u.

movement 10:
Draw from the Inexhaustible Source

Common Tai Chi Name: Stir the Whirlpool
This movement literally stirs the energy pool as the hands circle in horizontal motion together.

a. Withdraw your left arm to the rear and your right arm forward. Extend both arms with palms down. Elbows should not be locked.

b. While remaining in a Cat stance, circle the right hand across the torso to meet the left hand, which is extended out to the left side.

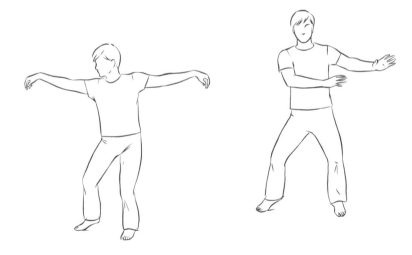

a.

b.

c. Now, from the left side, circle both hands out and clockwise, making a wide circle across the torso (whirlpool), turning palms down. As the arms circle to the right (through the level of the middle *tan tien*), set the right foot down to form a Bow stance facing the right and transfer 80 percent of your weight to the right foot.

d. Turn the palms up and circle them down toward the lower *tan tien*, moving back across your torso, close to your body, and ending on the left side. At the same time, shift your weight to the left foot and bring the right foot next to the left heel.

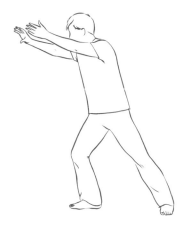

c.

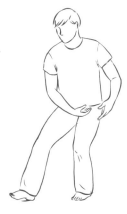

d.

movement 11:

The Feminine Yin Can Overcome the Masculine Yang

Common Tai Chi Name: Needle at the Bottom of the Sea
This movement draws energy from the lower and brings it to the upper. The left hand reaches deep as if grasping down a well.

a. Step the right foot onto the right rear diagonal and step the left foot close to the right foot to form a Half-Step. Eighty percent of your weight should now be on the right foot. At the same time, turn the left palm down, and push the left arm, slightly bent at the elbow, down to hover a foot above the knees. As you do this, begin to bend in the knees. The right elbow tucks into the crook of the left elbow, right palm up beside the left cheek.

b. Your arms stay in the same position, held together where right outer forearm meets left inner elbow, as you turn with the torso to the right. Continue to gently bring your arms around with the torso until your left forearm, still cradling your right arm, is hovering an inch above and across your right knee. Deeply bend the knees and keep your back straight. You are still holding most of your weight on your right foot.

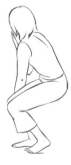

a.

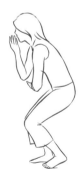

b.

movement 12:
Straight but Not Offensive

Common Tai Chi Name: Diagonal Flying
In this movement the left arm draws out and up toward the sky, then spirals in a continuous circle as the waist turns in a Twist stance, ending the spiral by rooting back down to the earth.

a. Straighten up as you step out to the side with the left foot onto the left front diagonal, facing your foot out at a forty-five-degree angle. Transfer your weight to the left foot and, as you do so, rotate your right foot (pivot on the heel) to the front. At the same time, pull your left hand from your right side to your left, turn your left palm up as you brush it past the right palm, which is facing down. Extend the left arm upward and outward to about face level, circling out counterclockwise while extending the right arm to the right side to about hip level.

b. Then step your right foot in a tiny bit toward your left, coming into a Horse stance and transfer your weight evenly on both feet. Rotate your body to the left while rotating the left foot outward (pivoting on the heel). Continue brushing arms outward until they balance evenly at shoulder level.

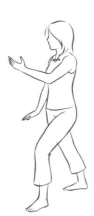

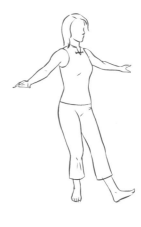

a.

b.

c. Continue pivoting on your left heel and your right ball until you have turned a full 180 degrees to face backward so that your right knee goes under your left knee. Set your left foot flat on the ground and transfer your weight to it. Your arms circle around with your rotating body, out to the sides like bird wings.

d. As your body twists to face the rear, cross your right arm in front of your left arm and bring them both together at the wrists. The palms should be facing outward to the sides, and your crossed arms should be in front of the middle *tan tien*. Bend your knees to a degree that is comfortable (raising your right heel if necessary) and keep your back straight.

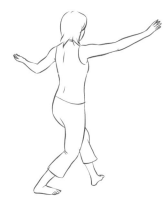

c.

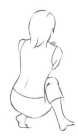

d.

movement 13:
To Be Brave Is to Be Kind

Common Tai Chi Name: Twist One Step Fist
This movement circles the energy out from the crouched earth position you took in movement 12 and prepares you for an expression of the yang virtue of courage.

a. From the previous position, stand up and straighten your still twisted knees (but do not fully extend), and let your hands descend, palms up. Curve your right hand gently down in front of your torso at the level of the lower *tan tien* as you bring your left hand out to the side, eventually falling down six inches away from the left hip. Your weight is still on your left leg.

b. Lift your right foot and step it out to the right, setting it down and pivoting around to the right on the right heel, with most of your weight on the right leg, and pivoting as well on the ball of your left foot, coming into a Twist stance while your body and arms begin to swing out to the right.

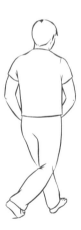
a.

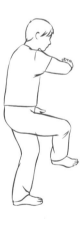
b.

c. Transfer the weight to your right foot. As your arms continue to swing to the right, bring the left hand, palm up, past the right hip and the right palm to face forward, away from the body, at shoulder height.

d. Continue to twist to the right and raise your left arm to shoulder height, while lowering your right hand out to the side to form a fist as you bring the left foot close to the right heel to form a Half-Step stance. Bring your right hand from out on the side to next to your right hip.

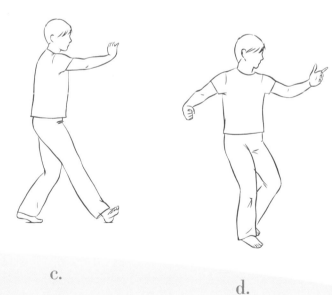

c.

d.

movement 14:
Within There Is Essence

Common Tai Chi Name: Move Block Fist
This movement asks for a forward fist punch, but one that's done in a gentle, nonaggressive manner consistent with the tai chi principle to "conserve energy within and not overextend without."

a. Step forward with the left foot and turn your right fist palm up. At the same time, turn the left hand palm down and lower it toward the right fist.

b. Turn the right fist into a vertical position as the left palm nears the right hip, and bring the left palm near the top of the right wrist. Turn the body forward and extend the right fist forward with the left hand resting on top of the right wrist no farther forward than the left knee.

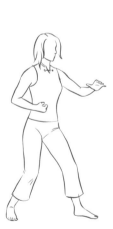

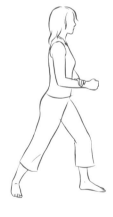

b.

a.

movement 15:
To Know When to Stop Is to Be Safe

Common Tai Chi Name: Withdraw and Push
In this movement you transition from a fist punch to a forward push with your hands circling horizontally at chest level. Again, the push never extends beyond the vertical plane of your knees, thereby preserving balance and security.

a. From the left Bow stance, rock more of your weight forward on the left foot and lift the right heel. Release your left hand from your right wrist.

b. Shift your weight back to the right leg and form a left Cat stance. At the same time, tuck your left hand under your right armpit and sweep it forward under the right arm to the right elbow. When the left arm reaches the right elbow, open your right fist so now both palms face up.

c. Sweep your left hand forward, coming under the right hand. When the left hand reaches the right hand, cross your hands at the wrist, left over right, with the palms facing your body, and bend your elbows so your hands are at chest level. Separate your hands to the sides in a horizontal circling motion.

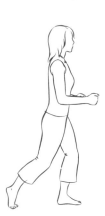

a.

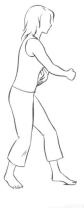

b.

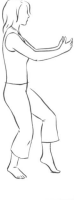

c.

d. Circle your hands in toward the middle *tan tien*. As your hands come in toward the chest, turn your palms to face outward. Step out with your left foot to form a Heel stance.

e. Place your left foot flat and come into a Bow stance as you push your hands forward. Your hands should not extend beyond the front knee.

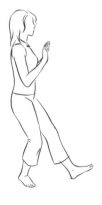

d.

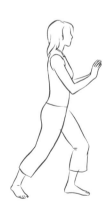

e.

movement 16:
Move without Exhaustion

Common Tai Chi Name: Fixed Step Cloud Hands
This movement is classically called "cloud hands" because it mimics the nature of the clouds floating in the sky without care, never exhausting themselves.

a. Begin by shifting your entire body to your right. From the left Bow stance, rotate your right flat foot to the front, transferring your weight to it. Rotate your torso to the right until you are facing front. Then bring your left foot back into a Horse stance facing the front as your left hand falls to your left side and your right arm sweeps across your body from left to right.

b. When in the Horse stance, turn your body to the right front diagonal and circle your right hand upward to shoulder level with palm down (your elbow should be lower than your wrist), while at the same time turning your left hand palm up and as it drops to the lower *tan tien*. Both hands should now be positioned as if holding a "ball" of energy. As you move, shift 60 percent of your weight to the right foot.

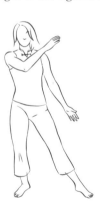

a.

b.

c. Turn your body to face the left front diagonal as you circle the left hand outward to the left and up to shoulder level with palm down (your elbow should be lower than your wrist), while at the same time turning your right hand palm up and bring it to the lower *tan tien*. As you move, shift 60 percent of your weight to the left foot. Repeat b and c two more times.

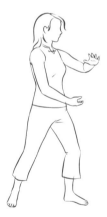

c.

movement 17:
Always Embrace the Source

Common Tai Chi Name: Cross Hands

This movement signifies the end of the routine as you gather energy and essence from all around. The heavenly and earthly energies are the source of our birth and existence.

a. From the previous position, turn your body to face front. While the left hand is still up, bring the right arm up to the level of the left arm. Turn your left arm to face outward and the right arm to face the torso.

b. Pull the arms apart at shoulder level, each out to the side, palms facing out. Your feet are still in Horse stance.

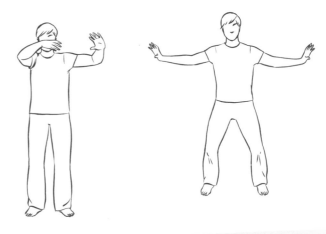

a.

b.

c. Then circle the arms outward and downward, bend at the knees, and swoop your arms downward as if you are scooping energy from the earth. Keep your back straight and your heels on the floor. Bend as far as is comfortable. At the bottom of the circle, cross your hands at the wrists, right over left.

d. Straighten up and bring your crossed hands up in front of the middle *tan tien*, with your palms facing your chest.

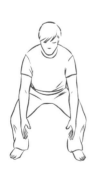

c.

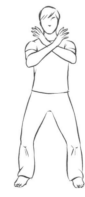

d.

movement 18:
Return to the Root

Common Tai Chi Name: Completion of Tai Chi
This is the last movement in 18-step harmony tai chi. Now that you have gathered the energy from outside of you, return that energy back to your root energy center, the *tan tien* in the lower abdomen.

a. From the previous position, uncross the hands and let them descend in front of the body toward the thighs.

b. Turn the hands palms up and circle them out to the sides and toward the front, with elbows bent, toward the level of the shoulders.

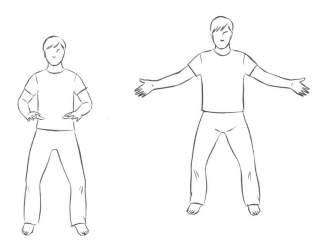

a.

b.

c. When the arms reach shoulder level, flip your palms over so they're now facing down. Let the arms descend slowly in front of the body toward the thighs with elbows bent.

d. Knees are still slightly bent as the hands reach toward the thighs.

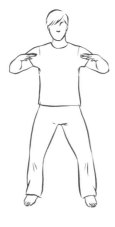

c.

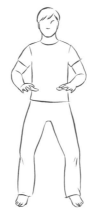

d.

movement 0:
The Great Void

Common Tai Chi Name: Wu Chi
Just as you started in an unmanifested state, you now return to the same state, completing a full circle.

Now let the hands move to the sides and straighten the knees slightly. The ending stance is the Great Void. The form ends where it begins. This embodies the principle that the manifested energy (yin and yang) of the Tao ultimately returns to the creative stillness of *wu chi*—the unmanifested subtle essence of the Tao.

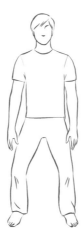

Closing Movement

a. When tai chi practice is finished, it is important to perform a closing movement in order to draw the expanded energy generated during tai chi practice back down into the lower *tan tien* for storage. This can be done in a Horse stance with knees slightly bent and arms down at the sides.

b. Slowly circle the arms outward and upward. When they reach the overhead position, palms should be facing downward.

c. Slowly let the arms descend (palms down) in front of the body toward the lower *tan tien*.

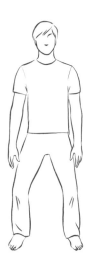

a.

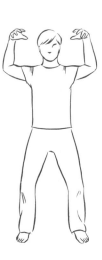

b.

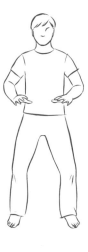

c.

d. When they reach the sides, circle the arms horizontally outward and toward the front at the level of the lower *tan tien*.

e. When the arms reach the front, palms should be facing toward the body. Then slowly bring the hands toward the lower *tan tien*. Stop when the palms are about twelve inches from the lower *tan tien*. Remain in this position for a few minutes.

continued on next page

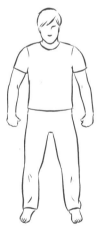
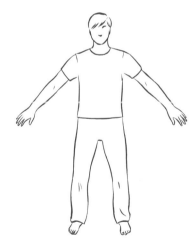
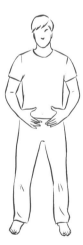

d.

e.

f. Then turn the palms downward and let the arms descend to the sides as the knees straighten and the feet come together.

BREATHING: As the arms circle outward and upward, inhale. As they descend, exhale. As the arms circle horizontally outward and toward the front, inhale. As they are drawn toward the lower *tan tien*, exhale. At all other times, breathe deeply and naturally.

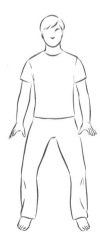

f.

continuing your tai chi practice

Deepening Your Practice

Initially, your focus will be on learning the movements and doing them correctly. Once you become familiar with the physical movements, you may go deeper in your practice, learning more subtle nuances of the Harmony Tai Chi form.

The external movements are the first level to master. By repeating them over and over, you will transmute your awkwardness into grace and sureness. Eventually, as you persist in your practice, you will become intimate with the cosmic law underlying the movements. Within the constant interplay of yin and yang, the complementary energies, you will find the absolute. Then, as you achieve true mastery, it will no longer be a limited, personal self who is practicing the movement: you will find that your entire life has merged with the universal energy.

As you devote yourself to your practice, you will find anything that furthers your spiritual self-cultivation to be relevant. For example, you might study acupuncture books to learn how energy flows through the meridians (or channels) of your body. Everything you learn will help you go deeper, beyond the mere physics of the movement, into the stillness of true self-discovery and awareness. By practicing regularly, you can achieve many states that cannot even be described in words.

Balancing Your Practice

We are all born with a natural tendency to be either right-handed or left-handed. The habit of depending on only one side of the body in daily activities, while neglecting the other side, creates or aggravates an imbalance. In order to correct such unbalanced development, qi practice offers us an opportunity to use both sides of our bodies.

For example, both my father and I are right-handed. When my father was small, he could not successfully use his left hand to cut the fingernails of his right with scissors. My grandmother suggested that he try to overcome this shortcoming, so he often switched hands when doing things. He learned to practice all of the tai chi movements beginning on the right side, as everybody did, but in his personal practice he would reverse the movements and begin them on the left. This means that all of the movements that were once to the right are now to the left and all the movements that were once to the left are now to the right. He usually stressed working with the left more than the right, because he already was using his right side in much of his daily life, and he felt that overall this would ultimately balance him, not just in practice, but in life.

Reversing the right side movements and doing them on the left side is not difficult. Generally, people have more strength on one side than the other, which is natural. However, to challenge yourself, pay special attention to your weaker side if you don't want it to remain clumsy.

When you have the time and ambition, try to practice your tai chi movements beginning with the left side on odd days and the right side on even days. Or try doing left movements in the morning and right movements in the afternoon, or vice versa. This routine is only one possibility. However you practice the physical arts, you should be flexible and never push yourself too hard. Your approach should always be in tune with your daily activities and life stage.

Achieving Self-Guidance

Harmony Tai Chi has a pure spiritual purpose: maintaining internal and external unity. Even after years and years of practice, you will not become tired of tai chi. Although you may expand your tai chi practice to encompass other forms, each will be like a special companion that enriches your life. Some forms are more suitable in certain types of weather, certain seasons, or certain times of day. When you achieve a certain level of practice, you will know which movements are best suited for specific situations.

All the movements can be adapted to your needs, depending only on your degree of self-awareness. You are not fixed by the form. From reading and from your own evolving spiritual insight, you can learn to personalize your practice for maximum benefit. Eventually, self-directed physical movement will become another component of your spiritual development.

Tai Chi Practice and **Reading**

When a student learns the form of tai chi from a teacher and stops there, his or her achievement will be limited. Cultivating your spiritual side by studying relevant texts will help you to continually fine-tune your tai chi practice.

Tai chi movement is based on the principle of harmony between the opposing forces of yin and yang; that also is the main theme of the *I Ching*. The gentle, unforced rhythms of movement and life are the essence of the *Tao Te Ching*. Both texts form a synergy with tai chi practice. The insights you gain from the movements will deepen your understanding of these books.

When you have a chance, try practicing tai chi in a garden while enjoying soothing music, a fragrant breeze, and the chirping of birds. Such special treats will replenish your spirit with pleasure and joy!

At the same time, as you develop in your practice, you will find that the most efficient way to nurture your own subtle energy is to refer regularly to the *I Ching* and the *Tao Te Ching*. You will be better equipped to correct your tai chi movements, and by continually deepening your understanding of these works, your tai chi movements will become more effective. Such deeper understanding also will help you improve your overall health, and it even can foster the subtle spiritual powers associated with immortality in China.

You might take half a year to read a short book like the *Tao Te Ching*, but after that six months, your awareness will be altered and improved. You will know intuitively how to correct your movements. You will penetrate beyond the surface of the form into its underlying structure and meaning.

Go Deeper Than the Form

In the beginning, when we choose to practice tai chi, we must become familiar with the basic form. We do this by practicing, and sometimes by watching and imitating others who are more experienced with tai chi. As our skills develop, the form itself will subtly change. As we progress, we will move to another, higher level.

The purpose of doing an exercise is not merely to imitate something already established. On the other hand, if people unfamiliar with tai chi even watch or imitate someone doing tai chi movements, they cannot help but notice fundamental principles of spiritual reality being manifested. They may not know it intellectually, but they will get a sense of it from watching or performing the movement themselves. Often beginners will become preoccupied with the surface qualities of a form and insist it can be done only a certain way. However, the real purpose of tai chi movement is to attain something not yet captured in any form.

We have to *start* with the form, because without it, we would have no way to learn. But our ultimate goal is a truth beyond any one form. People often ask me, "What is the Way?" meaning the path of tai chi. I have attempted to answer this question at different times, but my words speak only to the intellect. That is the nature of words. True, words can help our intellects glimpse the truth, but by patiently practicing and mastering tai chi, we can actually *become* the deep truth that underlies the movements.

Internalizing Tai Chi

The goal of Tai Chi is to attain harmony and balance. If we neglect the internal tai chi, our practice of tai chi will be like having the blueprint of a house we never build. Internal tai chi is a system that goes beneath or beyond the external form.

Once we have enough training and have practiced persistently, any movement we make can integrate our bodies, minds, and spirits. Even if we only think the words *tai chi*, we will immediately align ourselves in a balanced fashion. How do we do this? By deep practice. A Chinese proverb says, "When you learn to move, keep moving at all times. When you learn to sing, keep singing until you sing well." This means that when you learn tai chi movement, you should move your body as if you were doing tai chi movement all the time. That is how you will realize your true nature.

*con*clusion

The study of tai chi offers a rare opportunity for personal development. If we practice patiently and consistently, our skill and confidence will steadily grow. Both our material and spiritual goals will come into clearer focus, and we will be poised to savor the blessings of a long and contented life.

The most essential element of our practice is learning how to express our internal power effectively. In a practical sense, it is training ourselves in fear-lessness and life-affirming confidence.

Now that you have finished reading this book, the real fun begins. You can take the wisdom offered by tai chi and turn it into a dynamic self-reliance that animates everything you do. The consistent and determined practice of tai chi will bring you far more emotional and spiritual joy than movies or television or any of the usual diversions. Eventually, you will discover and experience the deep secrets of the universe as they unfold within this simple yet powerful cosmic dance. I invite you to tune in and start moving your life to the music of the primordial beat that resounds throughout time and space.

*re*sources

Harmony-Taichi.com

The official site of *Dr. Mao's Harmony Tai Chi*. The Web site provides further refinement and tips on the practice of Harmony Tai Chi short form as well as intermediate and long forms of Harmony Tai Chi. Information on other tai chi related forms, such as tai chi sword, can be found here. One can also view video clips of tai chi DVDs, search for scientific studies on the benefits of tai chi, look for a certified instructor near you, and subscribe to free e-mail newsletters.

www.harmony-taichi.com

Acupuncture.com

The oldest, most comprehensive, and most informative Web site on the Internet for acupuncture, Chinese herbal medicine, nutrition, tuina body work, tai chi, qigong, and related practices. This excellent resource for both consumers and practitioners offers access to hundreds of publications and herbal products.

www.acupuncture.com
info@acupuncture.com

Arthritis-Alternative.com

A Web site devoted to alternative methods of coping with arthritis, including tai chi—which has been confirmed through studies to be beneficial for arthritis sufferers. The Web site also features natural supplements and remedies for promoting healthy joints.

www.arthritis-alternative.com
info@arthritis-alternative.com

AskDrMao.com

The official Web site of Dr. Maoshing Ni's book *Secrets of Longevity*. The site features antiaging recipes, tools for healthy living, product reviews, and new tips for living a long, healthy, and happy life. You can also subscribe to free e-mail newsletters here.

www.askdrmao.com

Chi Health Institute (CHI)

CHI is a nonprofit association that is dedicated to promoting health through the Taoist movement arts as transmitted by the Ni Family. Inspired by the teachings of the Integral Way by the author's father, Master Ni Hua-Ching, the Institute offers professional level education and instructor certification programs for tai chi, qi gong, and meditation. The Web site also maintains a directory listing of certified instructors in Harmony tai chi and other movement arts.

13315 W. Washington Blvd., Suite 301
Los Angeles, CA 90066

www.chihealth.org

Healing People Network

Comprehensive Web site on complementary and alternative medicine (CAM) for consumers and practitioners. In-depth coverage of subjects such as acupuncture, aromatherapy, ayurveda, bodywork, Chinese medicine, cancer risk reduction, environmental toxicology, fitness training, herbalism, homeopathy, naturopathy, nutrition and lifestyle, pet health, and other natural healing modalities. The site also provides a referral network of CAM practitioners throughout the United States and access to more than 1,000 pharmaceutical-grade supplement products.

906 E. Verdugo Rd.
Burbank, CA 91501

www.healingpeople.com
contact@healingpeople.com

Integral Way Society

A nonprofit, community group founded by Mentors and students of the Integral Way tradition whose aim is to serve the modern world through sharing the natural wisdom of the tradition of Lao Tzu and the ancient Taoist sages as interpreted by Master Ni Hua-Ching. The Society promotes balance, health, harmony, and virtue through personal growth and spiritual development.

www.integralwaysociety.org
contact@integralwaysociety.org

SevenStar Communications Group

An excellent resource on Taoism, Eastern philosophy, and the Integral Way tradition that is the foundation of Harmony tai chi. The site features many previous books and audio/video titles from the author and his father, Master Ni Hua-Ching.

13315 W. Washington Blvd., Suite 201
Los Angeles, CA 90066

www.sevenstarcom.com
info@sevenstarcom.com

Tao of Wellness

Health and wellness centers in Southern California that specialize in providing quality service in acupuncture and Chinese medicine. Co-founded by Dr. Maoshing Ni, this is also where he sees patients in his group practice.

1131 Wilshire Blvd., Suite 300
Santa Monica, Ca 90401

www.taoofwellness.com
contact@taoofwellness.com

Yo San University of Traditional Chinese Medicine

An accredited graduate school of traditional Chinese medicine founded by Dr. Maoshing Ni and his family. Its rigorous academic, clinical, and spiritual development programs train students for the professional practice of acupuncture and Eastern medicine. Its unique Qi Development Program helps its students develop sensitivity and mastery of energy that are essential for practicing acupuncture and Chinese medicine.

13315 W. Washington Blvd., Suite 200
Los Angeles, CA 90066

www.yosan.edu
admissions@yosan.edu

*in*dex